Super Health For Super Kids

Parenting Guides For Picky Eating And Stronger Immune System

Jennifer schwarz

Copyright © Jennifer Schwarz, 2022

LEGAL NOTICE

The Publisher has strived to be as accurate and complete as possible in the creation of this report, notwithstanding the fact that he does not warrant or represent at any time that the contents within are accurate due to the rapidly changing nature of the Internet.

While all attempts have been made to verify information provided in this publication, the Publisher assumes no responsibility for errors, omissions, or contrary interpretation of the subject matter herein. Any perceived slights of specific persons, peoples, or organizations are unintentional.

In practical advice books, like anything else in life, there are no guarantees of income made. Readers are cautioned to reply on their own judgment about their individual circumstances to act accordingly.

This book is not intended for use as a source of legal, business, accounting or financial advice. All readers are advised to seek services of competent professionals in legal, business, accounting and finance fields.

You are encouraged to print this book for easy reading.

Table Of Contents

Forward

Chapter 1
  Introduction

Chapter 2
  What Children Require For A Healthful Diet

Chapter 3
  What Foods Should Children Avoid?

Chapter 4
  Simple Strategies To Encourage Children To Eat Healthfully

Chapter 5
  Exercise Needs for Children

Chapter 6
  Easy Exercise Activities For Children

Chapter 7
  The Effects of Stress on Children

Chapter 8
  How to Aid Children in De-Stressing

Chapter 9
  New Technologies in Pediatric Health

Chapter 10
  The Advantages Of Teaching Children About Health

Conclusion

Forward

One of the most significant responsibilities of parents is to protect their children's health. Teach your children the fundamentals of health while they are still young since many people nowadays live unhealthy and sedentary lifestyles. Learn all you need right here.

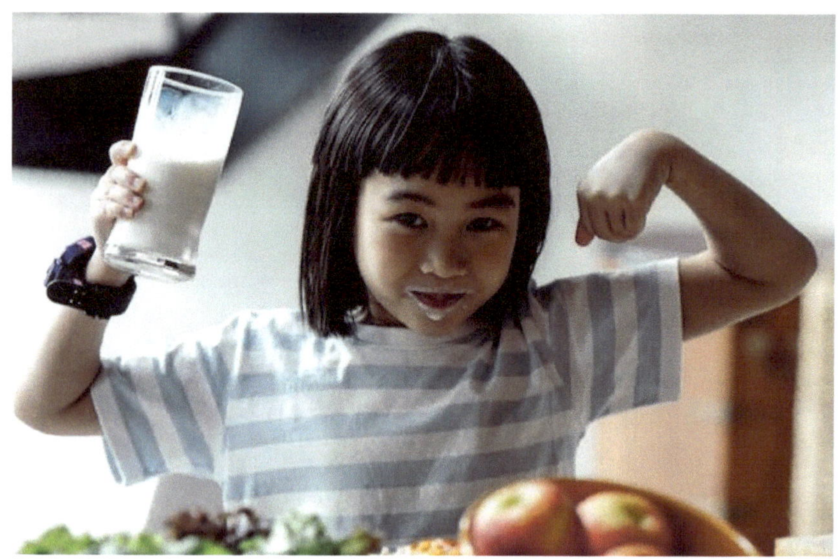

Chapter 1

Introduction

You need to assist them in understanding the many facets of their health while yet being able to advise them. You don't have to sound like you're delivering a sermon or lecture when doing this. You can ensure that your children have healthy, balanced lives by providing them with love and care in addition to their everyday activities.

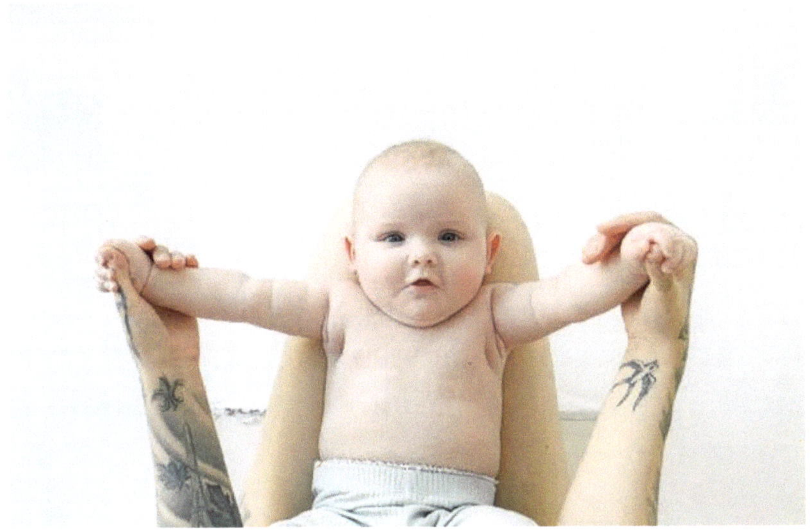

What Is Basic

Creating the Best Habits

The behaviors that children form will undoubtedly persist throughout adulthood. Every parent is responsible for assisting their children in developing healthy habits while they are still young. Along with character development, you should also examine your children's everyday routines, such as the foods they consume, their physical activity, their interactions with others, and their impressions of the world around them.

Little is known about the world to children. Most of the time, kids are easily seduced by meals or even activities that they see as entertaining and amusing without thinking about the harmful consequences.

You must discipline your children to develop into mature, responsible, health-conscious adults to support them.

Healthy Eating

When it comes to feeding their children, many parents, if not all, will encounter difficulties. After all, adults struggle to maintain a balanced diet, mostly because it requires them to consume wholesome but bland foods.

Children's appetites may be quite delicate. Young children are often readily persuaded to consume meals high in fat, such as fried chicken, French fries, etc. Numerous children cannot refuse to consume chocolates, sweets, and other foods high in sugar. There's nothing wrong with this.
However, anything in excess may also be harmful. You must watch what your children consume as a parent. You may use strategies to provide inventive meals that are tasty and nourishing.

Physical Exercise

Kids need to exercise in addition to their normal dietary routines. Given their advanced age, you cannot force them to exercise if they choose not to. You may make sure that your children are physically active by having them participate in sports or other activities that include playing with other children. Your youngster not only gets to socialize with other children but also has the opportunity to exercise covertly.

Learn a Lot of Advice from This Book

This EBook's primary goal is to provide a comprehensive strategy and illuminating advice for ensuring your children's health. The eBook is broken into many parts that address topics including stress, exercise, and a healthy diet. You have the opportunity to learn more about the many facets of your child's health with the help of these practical advice, recipes, and other crucial details.

Chapter 2

What Children Require For A Healthful Diet

You must be aware of the exact foods that your children must consume as well as the appropriate amounts of vitamins and minerals if you want to make sure that their diets are full and well-balanced.

The knowledge of what foods to consume and what meals to avoid is widespread among parents. But it's also important to understand the proper serving size to ensure you get all the vitamins and minerals your body needs.

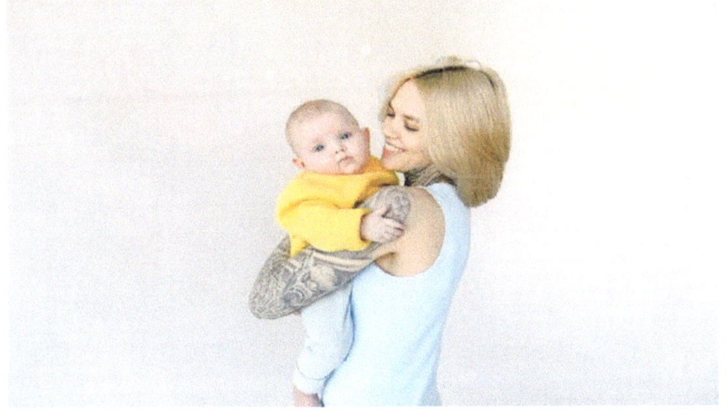

What They Need

Dietary Recommendations for Young Children and Toddlers

For growth and development, toddlers and young children need the full complement of nourishment. Knowing the dietary recommendations can help you as a parent prepare the correct meals for your children.

Whole grains: You may have buckwheat pancakes or toast in the morning. You may serve brown rice with supper at night. Just make sure your children have four servings of healthy grains each day.

Fruits And Vegetables: Your children should consume two servings of fruits and vegetables each day. You may eat an apple or other fruit-containing snacks in the morning. Additionally, you may make nutritious vegetable soups.

Protein: Children need protein to help their muscles grow. You need two servings each day. Encourage your children to consume baked beans, eggs, lamb, fish, and lamb.

Milk And Dairy: Three servings of milk and dairy products must be given to your child daily for proper bone formation. Your child is welcome to have cheese, milk, yogurt, etc.

Minerals and vitamins: Taking supplements may also assist in ensuring that your children get the appropriate dosage of minerals and vitamins.

Nutritional Advice for Children in School

As children mature, they will need to consume more and get the nourishment that adults need. Along with fruits, vegetables, nutritious proteins, and whole grains like oats, rice, and millet, your children also need to consume healthy fats, which include the following:

Monounsaturated fats: sesame seeds, avocados, canola oil, and peanut oil.

Crackers, cookies, margarine, and other foods contain **Trans Fats**.

Polyunsaturated: Omega 3 fatty acids are healthy for the heart, and Omega 6 fatty acids are found in foods like salmon, sardines, anchovies, walnuts, and many more.

Dietary Suggestions

Whole Grains: Children in school-age groups should consume 6 to 11 servings of whole grains daily.

Fruits: You should offer 2-4 servings of fruits per day, which may be either sliced fruit or 34 cups of any fruit juice.

Vegetables: Three to five servings of vegetables are required daily. One cup of leafy vegetables or 3/5 cups of vegetable juice may be served.

Dairy Products: 2-3 servings of yogurt, milk, or natural cheese.

Zinc: Zinc, which is included in many foods, including beef, hog, liver, milk, cocoa, and chicken, is necessary to improve memory and academic performance.

Prepare delicious and nourishing meals.

Getting your child to eat nutritious meals might be difficult, particularly if they have delicate tastes in cuisine. Be inventive in the meals you create, and always remember that you should produce delectable meals if you want to guarantee a full intake of vitamins and minerals.

Chapter 3

What Foods Should Children Avoid?

Kids like desserts and other unhealthful foods. Knowing which foods to avoid is crucial since your kids' eating might affect their growth and development. You may assist your children with their eating habits by letting them know which foods and meals to steer clear of.

Of course, it is impossible to always watch over your children, particularly at school. However, you must assist children in forming healthy eating habits while they are still young.

Do Not Approach These

Limit Sugar

Every one of us has memories of consuming various sweets and chocolates as a youngster. When kids enjoy these delectable sweets and decadent chocolates, they are happiest. There is nothing wrong with letting your children consume sweets. However, you should watch out, so they don't go overboard. The American Heart Association recommends that youngsters consume no more than 12 grams or three teaspoons daily.

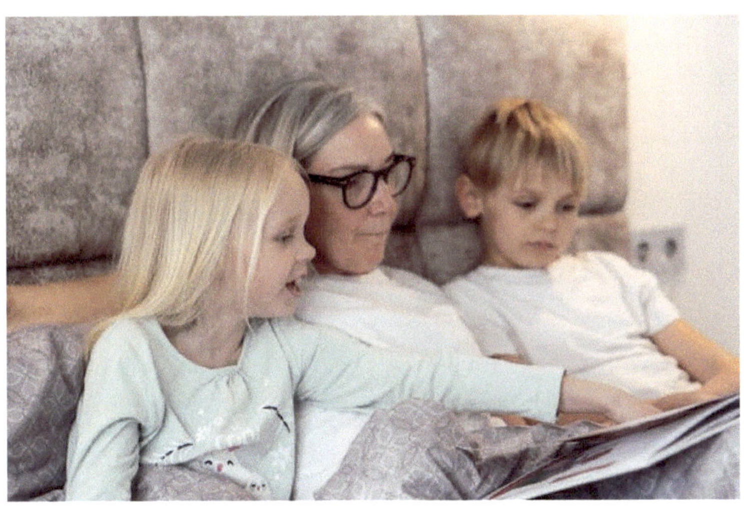

You may decrease your sugar consumption in some ways. One benefit is that you can cook and prepare dishes with less sugar. Avoiding sugary beverages like soft drinks and sodas is another alternative. You may swap these beverages out for wholesome smoothies. Last but not least, avoid giving processed meals to your children.

Reduce Salt-Containing Products Consumption

The body also needs sodium. Kids, however, cannot consume too much salt. 2,300 mg of sodium are already present in one teaspoon of salt. There are recommendations regarding the maximum amount of salt that young children should consume. The recommended daily salt intake for children aged 1 to 3 is 1,500 mg. Children between the ages of 4 and 8 should not exceed 1,900 mg of salt per day. The daily salt limit for children aged 9 to 13 is 2,200 mg.

How do you control how much salt they eat?

There are several strategies to consume less salt. Today's youth just like dining out and consuming fast food. Most of these businesses employ excessive salt levels. It is highly advised that you make meals at home rather than eat at fast food places if you want to reduce your salt intake.

Additionally, eating fresh veggies rather than those in cans was advised. You must pick low-salt foods when you shop.

Don't Consume Junk Foods

Junk food is widely available. Your children would undoubtedly like consuming various junk foods. These goods are nutritionally deficient; some even have excessive salt and sugar content. As a result, you must advise your children to abstain from consuming junk food or, if that is not feasible, to limit their intake.

Alternatives that are healthier options abound. For instance, your kids could choose graham crackers, fruit dips, bagels, or English muffins over potato chips. Your children may choose low-fat frozen yogurt or fruit smoothies over ice cream.

Chapter 4

Simple Strategies To Encourage Children To Eat Healthfully

Since they need certain vitamins and minerals to help them develop, children should eat a nutritious diet. They may further improve their bodies, sharpen their brains, and become more physically energized and active with the appropriate sort of nutrition.

Unfortunately, many parents struggle with various issues in this area, making it easier said than done. Children still need to be taught which foods are healthy and which are not, for one thing. Second, most youngsters are naturally inclined to like consuming items like chocolates and sweets high in sugar. Thirdly, kids prefer unhealthy meals like fast food and other greasy food items, which is a natural part of their youth.

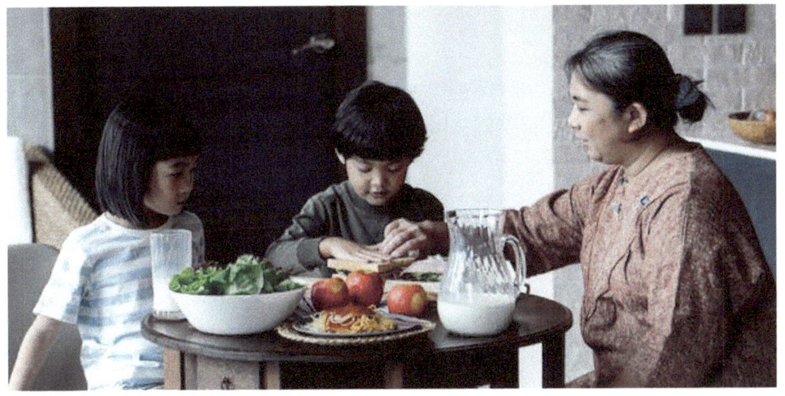

Take the simple route.

Create Healthy Eating Habits

You must assist children in forming healthy eating habits. You can still let your kids consume foods like chocolates and fried chicken. However, you must ensure kids consume more nutrient-dense meals and get all the vitamins and minerals their bodies need.

How precisely do you mold their eating behaviors?

- Eat meals at home often. Children need to understand when and what to eat during meals. When you prepare meals at home, you can be sure that the components are nutritious, as opposed to letting your children consume fast food or purchasing food from the canteen. Prepare meals at home so you can keep an eye on what they're eating.

- Permit them to take part. Children want to participate as well. You may take your kids with you to the grocery store and let them choose what they want in their lunchbox. Simply keep an eye on their choices, sort them out, and explain why they should steer clear of harmful food items.

- Prepare wholesome yet nourishing meals. Kids dislike eating healthy meals for various reasons, but one of the primary ones is that some people make bland, unattractive food. You may look for recipes to entice your kids to eat nutritious meals. Online, where you can cook nutrient-dense meals without sacrificing flavor. When preparing any dish, use your imagination. To make a dish more aesthetically pleasing, you could wish to utilize certain artistic approaches.

- Encourage children to consume more produce, especially fruits. You may make tasty smoothies every morning that your kids will undoubtedly like. Additionally, people might eat vegetables in various meals without realizing it.

- Serve meals in moderate amounts. Over the years, there has been an increase in the number of children who are obese. If ignored, this might become a major issue. You should always offer the proper quantity of every meal to prevent dealing with this issue. If you observe that your children tend to eat more than a typical child, you should give appetite control significant thought to prevent weight gain.

Chapter 5

Exercise Needs for Children

Kids need to exercise just as adults do. In addition to the value of social interaction and interaction with others, children who engage in regular physical activity improve their physical health.

Since most children like playing and being active, encouraging them to exercise is not particularly tough. They like playing with other kids and running about. These physical activities qualify as an exercise by themselves.

Your children may experiment with various workouts and games. They may choose whatever activity they wish, based on their preferences.

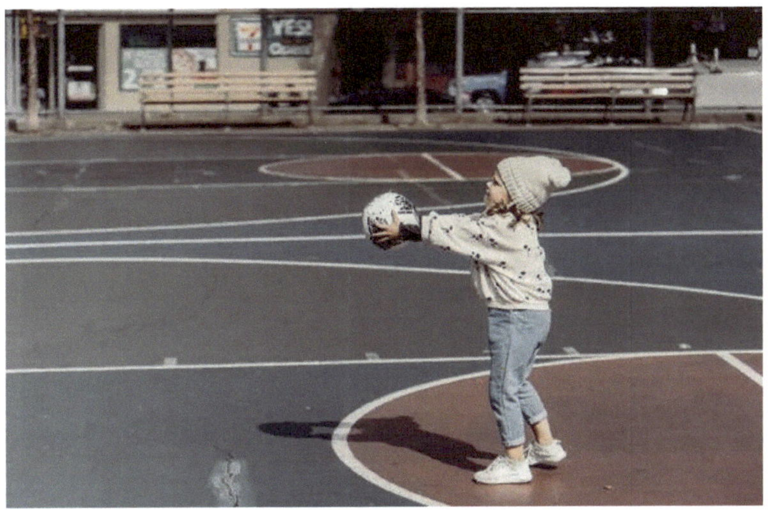

Exercise

Motivation's Vitality

Since most children are active, it only seems sensible that they would choose to play most of the time. However, some kids have pretty distinct personalities as well. Some people would like to remain home and engage in things that don't require a lot of physical activity.

When this occurs, kids need to practice motivation as soon as possible. This is also one of the hardest things to accomplish, mainly if the children show no interest. However, parents may discover methods to encourage their children to exercise if they are patient.

Scheduling Exercise Time

Parents should monitor their children's daily routines and ensure time is set aside for exercise while they are occupied with schoolwork and other obligations. Your children may exercise by setting aside an hour each day for it.

Other physical activities and sports

One of the best forms of exercise for your children is playing sports. They not only help a person acquire self-control but also their general health. You may sign up your child for a taekwondo class or any activity that piques his interest. Before him

You should get him the supplies he needs, such as his taekwondo costume before he starts the lesson.

You may consider enrolling your child in a ballet

lesson or a skating program for females. Children who are enrolled in a skating lesson must have the appropriate attire in addition to their ice skates. Children taking dance classes need to wear dance shoes. They may perform better and enjoy their lessons more when dressed appropriately.

Your child's interest should always be the primary factor taken into account when choosing an activity. What activities do they like doing?

Equipment and Tools

Several physical activities may call for specific tools and gear. Children may desire to attempt other sports like cycling, ice hockey, or any activity that requires certain instruments and equipment. Parents of kids who are passionate about these hobbies should unquestionably encourage them. These pastimes could advance later, and youngsters might begin to discover their love.

Parents must invest in their children. Even if you may have to spend some money only to make sure they focus on improving their physical health, at least you get to meet your children's requirements.

Of course, there are other, less expensive methods for kids to exercise.

Chapter 6

Easy Exercise Activities For Children

Regular exercise is also necessary for children to develop the many facets of their health. Children are, by nature, lively and fun, which makes sense given that youth is characterized by energy. As a result, you won't have any problems with this. They already have the opportunity to exercise when they run about and play with other children.

On the other hand, some youngsters aren't as active as others. Other children are pretty shy and don't really like physical activities. Some children choose to participate in activities other than exercise.

If so, parents should discover strategies to encourage their children to exercise. This may be difficult if your youngster doesn't want to participate in a lot of physical activity.

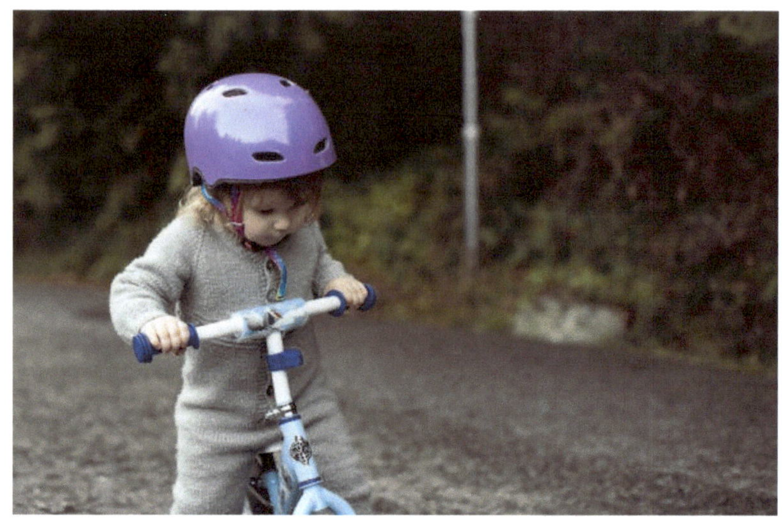

Make Them Move

What steps should you take?

1. Embrace their socialization.

You don't have to coerce children into following the typical adult fitness regimens to persuade them to exercise. Many children like playing in parks and playgrounds. Even if your child isn't active physically, they can still play with other kids. It already counts as exercise since he is playing with his pals. Running about and having fun with other kids is the most fun.

2. Encourage kids to take up sports.

Any sport is open to people of all ages. Depending on their preferences, even children may attempt various sports. They may choose the specific sport they wish to attempt, such as swimming, taekwondo, table tennis, or skating.

When children participate in sports, there are several advantages. This is the ideal type of exercise, particularly for kids who attempt extreme physical activities like jogging, swimming, judo, and taekwondo. Second, playing sports may help youngsters learn responsibility. As kids become older, they become more responsible. Sports aid in a child's personality and character development. This is a major factor in why many parents desire to sign up their children for various sporting activities.

3. To make physical activities more enjoyable, parents should participate with their kids.

Parents are welcome to participate in any physical activity their kids engage in. Children are more encouraged to play when they witness their parents playing with them. Additionally, parents are allowed to connect and spend time with their children. You may arrange various weekend activities for your kids and watch them enjoy themselves. You may do several activities with your children that will allow them to move their bodies.

4. Try some indoor pursuits

There are indoor hobbies that young people might do if they truly don't want to go outside too often. Children may walk around and exercise while playing on gaming consoles. Parents may also spend money on various tools and equipment so that children can exercise even while at home.

Chapter 7

The Effects of Stress on Children

One of the main causes of why so many individuals get certain illnesses and diseases is stress. Kids are not immune to stress, even if adults are more likely to encounter it owing to employment, lifestyle, and interpersonal interactions. A variety of circumstances may cause stress. Children may feel stress at home or even at school.

Protecting your children from stressful circumstances is challenging, given the complex interactions individuals have nowadays and the environment they live in. Therefore, parents must try to prevent their children from experiencing stress.

Stress may have a detrimental effect on a child's behavior and even how they see the world. How do children react to stress?

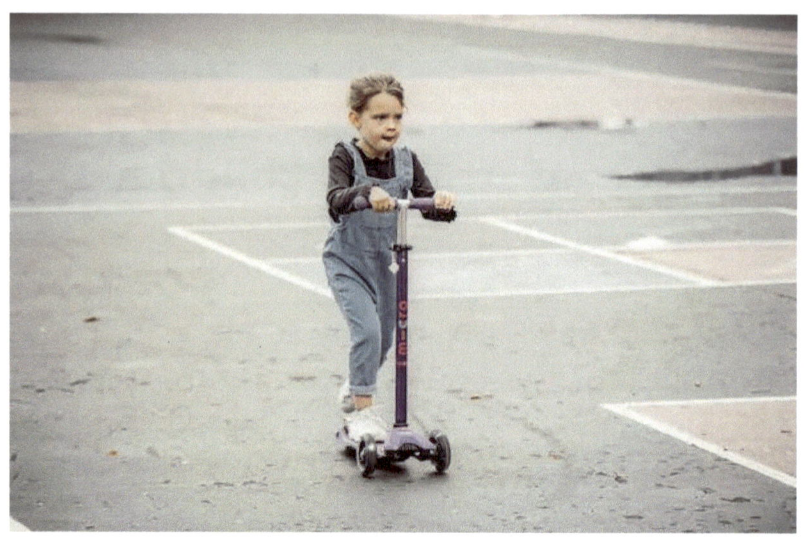

Children And Stress

1. Children's mental development is impacted by stress.

According to research, children who face stressful circumstances are more likely to have issues with their mental development. Children have difficulties when they are anxious. Children struggle to focus in school on their subjects. Their ability to concentrate may also be hampered, which may negatively impact their academic performance in general.

2. Children's conduct may be substantially altered by stress

Stress at home and school tends to cause children to behave very differently. One of the most obvious effects is that children who experience significant stress tend to isolate themselves and become distant. They often lack self-confidence and shy away from interpersonal interactions.

Low self-esteem may occur in certain children who face stressful circumstances. This has an impact on their self-perception and interactions with others.

3. Their eating habits may be impacted by stress

You must provide your child meals that are fully nutrient-dense to ensure their growth and development. Along with feeding them nutritious food, you should also take steps to prevent stress in the house for your children. An anxious child's eating patterns could alter. Some kids tend to overeat, which may eventually lead to obesity, while other youngsters may lose their appetite and refuse to eat.

This will significantly impact their overall growth and development. Kids may encounter health issues and other health hazards if they don't have a balanced diet without added stress.

4. How Can Children Reduce Stress?

Children are protected by their families and other loved ones, unlike adults who must live and face the world alone. Despite their innocence and youth, kids shouldn't be exposed to stressful events that may negatively impact their attitude, conduct, and even character.

Your responsibility as a parent is to ensure that your children are raised in a calm, safe, and stress-free atmosphere. Of course, it is impossible to completely avoid stressful circumstances. But while your children are still little, you should do everything you can to shelter and protect them. After all, they are mostly ignorant of the complex issues surrounding them.

Chapter 8

How to Aid Children in De-Stressing

At some time in their lives, children may feel stressed. Both parents and children cannot escape this. For instance, it may be distressing for a child to see his parents fighting or bickering. Children who struggle in school may also get stressed.

Parents can't shield their children completely from difficult events. However, parents may assist by finding methods to relieve their children's tension. It's critical for children who experience stress to have a solid support system.

What can you do to relieve your children's stress in various ways?

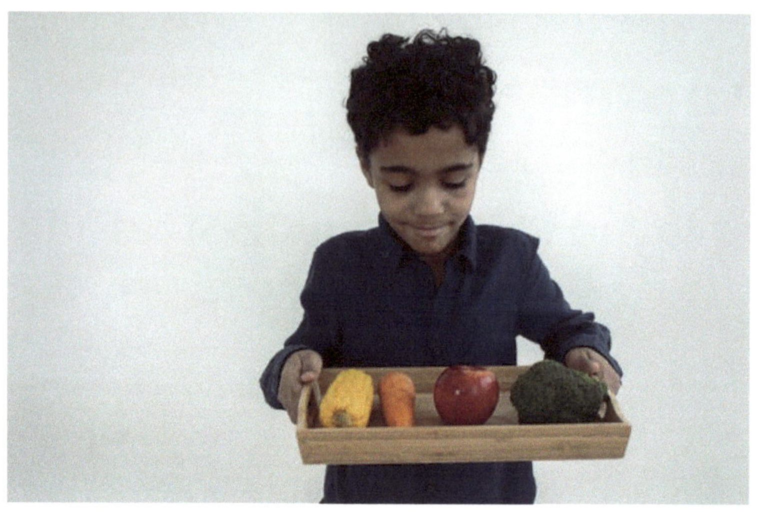

How To Assist

1. Communication's Vitality

Due to their busy schedules and other responsibilities, many parents often overlook the need for communication. Some parents hardly take the time to inquire about their children's well-being, despite attending to their necessities. Children may feel alone if there is no interaction or dialogue. When anything awful occurs, or they are put in a stressful scenario, they will undoubtedly find it difficult to deal with the issue. They do not wish to divulge it to anybody else.

That is why it is so important for parents to talk to their children all the time. Children may express their emotions and opinions to their parents when they chat. They do not have to bear the weight alone if they experience any stress. Undoubtedly, their parents can soothe them.

2. Schedule time for your children

Family relationships are crucial, particularly for children who go through developmental periods when they may encounter challenging circumstances that they find very stressful. Children must not feel alone in their journey; this must be a priority.

Parents should constantly demonstrate to their children how much they value and care for them. You should constantly try to interact and communicate with your children regardless of how busy you are. You should find time in your hectic schedule to spend quality time with your children and demonstrate their importance to you. Youngsters who experience love at home may easily get through challenging circumstances.

3. Protect your health

You must ensure that your children's requirements are met, particularly those related to their general health, if you want them to be active and lively at school. Prepare nourishing meals to increase their energy and sharpen their intellect. Kids who eat balanced meals and get the recommended vitamins and minerals daily are less likely to experience stress.

Complete sleep is another crucial element. Youngsters tend to get quickly agitated when they don't get nearly enough sleep. Make sure your children get a full night's sleep by putting them to bed early.

4. Under Pressure Grace

Children often mimic what they observe. Children's attitudes regarding clothing might be influenced by their parent's actions and attitudes toward certain occasions or events. Because of this, parents must always act graciously when they are faced with challenging circumstances.

Chapter 9

New Technologies in Pediatric Health

Significant changes have been brought about by technology for both adults and children. When you visit various places, you'll see a huge selection of contemporary goods your kids would undoubtedly adore and appreciate. There are other areas of your child's growth and development where the technology may be a helpful contributing component, apart from simply the entertainment value it can provide.

How can you utilize the current technology to enhance the general health of your children in the context of new technology and health? Can technology truly be used to improve the health of children?

The answer is undoubtedly a resounding yes!

There are now options for improving the many facets of your children's health thanks to technological breakthroughs. The following would be some of these:

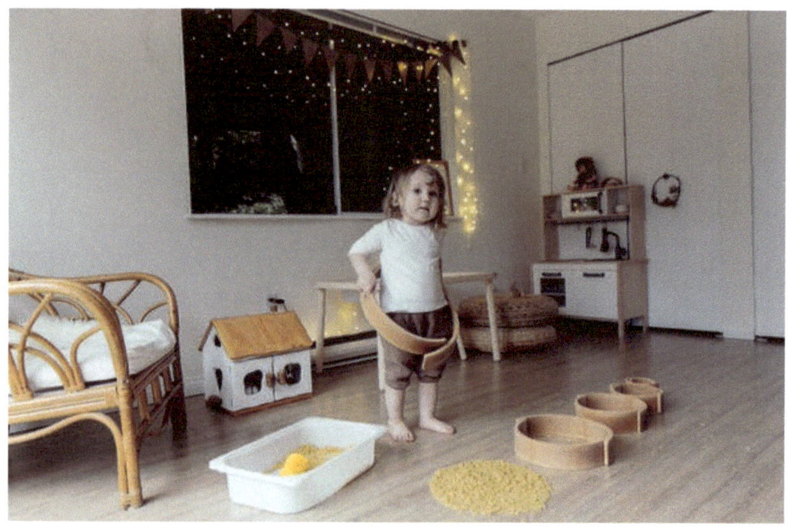

New Technology

Mental Wellness

The improvement of your mental health is one of the areas that you can do using technology. Many children nowadays are more clever and competitive. They have no trouble using various tools and technologies. Now is the moment for parents to use modern technologies.

For instance, parents might let their children play various internet games to improve their memory and expand their imaginations. Children may play various games on a portable device that requires them to exercise their minds and devise tactics. They may converse and socialize with other youngsters who are playing the same game, in addition to that.

Parents should still supervise their children anytime they use these devices for educational reasons.

Physical Fitness

Physical health is another area of health that may be improved with the aid of technology. Kids may simply choose the precise things they wish to own to enhance their physical health since so many products are accessible to them.

Children may now play video games on gadgets that allow them to walk about and exercise. Due to gaming gadgets, they may dance and participate in other sports without leaving their homes. Not only do kids enjoy themselves, but they may also exercise without even realizing it.

Oral Fitness

Simply said, children adore sweets. It is difficult to restrain their sweet tooth from anything from candy to chocolate. While parents can keep an eye on what their kids eat, there are certain situations when it is impossible for them to. As a consequence, some children—if not all—suffer from serious oral health issues. Some people could get dental decay.

However, owing to technology, there are now a variety of dental services available in addition to the many dental treatments and procedures to guarantee that your children will have a full set of pearly-white teeth. Dentists now employ modern technologies to assist youngsters in maintaining healthy teeth and preventing tooth decay.

Chapter 10

The Advantages Of Teaching Children About Health

You may start laying the groundwork for guaranteeing your children's health very early. Even if they may not entirely comprehend what you want to achieve, you still have the opportunity to lead them. Little doubt that the meals kids consume may affect their overall growth and development.

As a parent, you may raise your children, so they get the proper nourishment and a safe, healthy environment in which to develop. There are long-term advantages to educating children about healthy health.

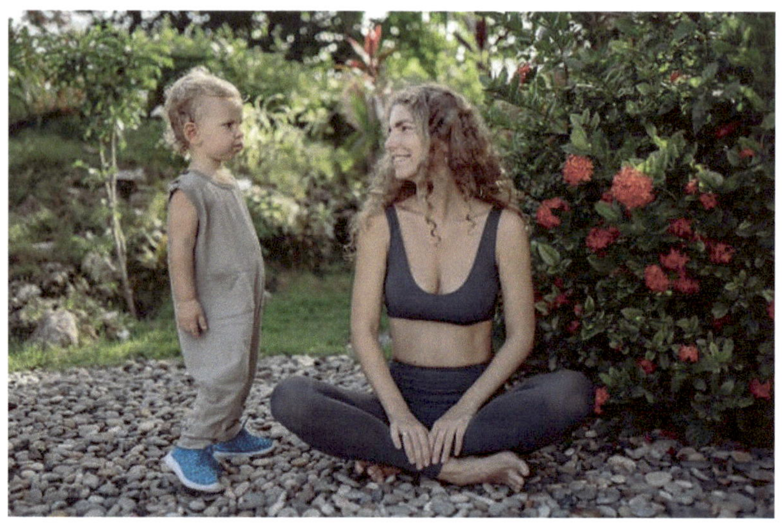

The Benefits

1. They form the proper habits.

Adults who have sedentary lifestyles often have poor eating habits. In addition to not exercising, some like eating meals high in fat, salt, and sugar. Some people might smoke or drink. These are all largely attributable to the habits they were able to form while still very young.

This is one of the causes why youngsters must start developing positive behaviors while still young. For instance, you should restrict the meals your children eat to those that are nutritious. Children who choose to eat fruits and veggies will continue to practice these healthy behaviors as they age.

2. You watch over the growth and development of your child.

The appropriate behaviors for your child to grow are simply one part. When parents stress the value of health, they also safeguard their children's growth. Kids' diets may have a beneficial or negative effect on their development. The development of children may be badly impacted if parents let their children eat anything they want without ensuring they are getting all the necessary nutrients.

3. You establish the fundamentals and requirements for optimal health.

You also establish the groundwork for excellent health by teaching your children healthy food practices. One blatant example is that if your child begins participating in sports at a young age, he or she will be able to maintain that attitude in the future. Therefore, It is generally advised that parents should truly encourage their children to engage in their preferred sports if they enjoy such games.

4. Children may make difficult situations diminish.

When a child is healthy, he or she is less likely to experience stress than other children. Remember that the foods your children consume, their everyday interactions, and their hobbies might cause stress. However, if your child consumes nourishing meals and regular exercises, stress should be something they can easily avoid.

Conclusion

Long-term advantages might result from assisting your child in forming healthy behaviors and laying the groundwork for investigating their overall health. Your responsibility and duty as a parent are to offer your children the greatest possible life. At least your child will always remember what you taught him/her as they become older and start to grow up.

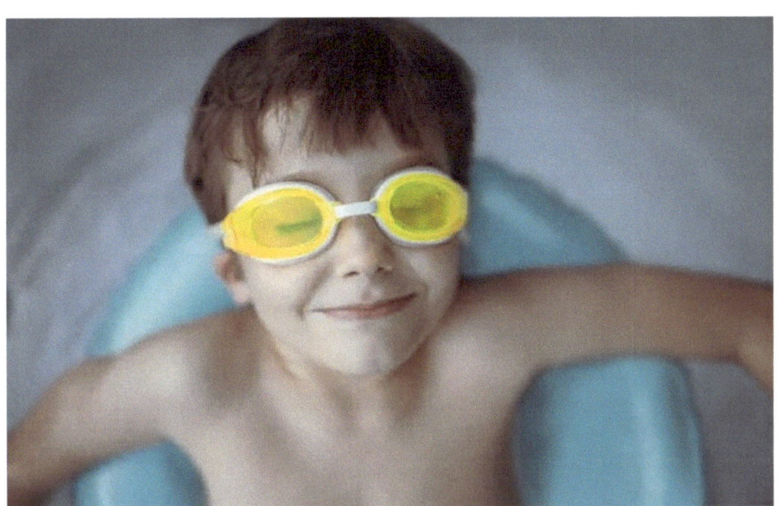